This Way to Florida

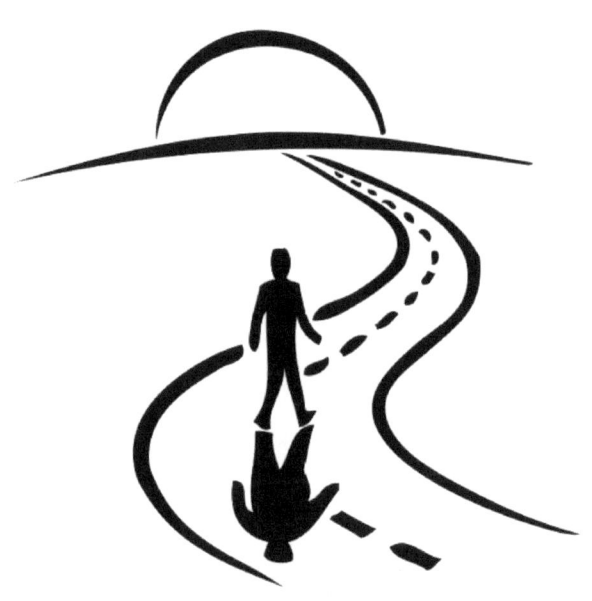

This Way to Florida

—ɯ—

A Prescription for Weight Loss

Steven R. Uttley, MD

ISBN 10: 1514861461
ISBN 13: 9781514861462
Library of Congress Control Number: 2015910871
CreateSpace Independent Publishing Platform
North Charleston, South Carolina

Acknowledgments

First, I have to thank my close friend and colleague Dr. Michael Crouzat for his advice and especially for his design of the logo for my book cover and for the This Way diet plan.

Starting a weight-loss program, sticking with it, and eventually reaping the reward require a lot of support. I could not have done it during the nearly two years from the start of this journey without the support of my partner Dr. Ginette Rainville through medical school, residency, the army, my heart surgery, and beyond. I also have to thank my cousin and athlete Marc Lamothe for his motivation, inspiration, advice and encouragement along the way. This project would not have seen the light of day without him.

The encouragement I get from my friends, staff, and patients who have noticed my transformation is also priceless. And thanks to you for buying this book and supporting my efforts to get the word out about weight loss and the fact that anyone can do it by sticking to a plan. This is the one that worked for me.

Disclaimer

Before you attempt this program, please check with your doctor. This program is not for everyone. It is what worked for me at my level of health. If you have any serious or chronic medical conditions, such as diabetes or heart disease, you should consult your doctor to ensure that the dietary plan and exercise are OK for you. I individualize this program for patients in my office, so only your doctor can approve this program for you—unless, of course, I am your doctor.

Introduction

The first step in achieving anything is literally the first step. You couldn't walk until the day you took your first one. It was not easy, and for the most part, it was a long time coming. For most people, the ability to walk as a child comes after about a year of development. It takes some time for the nervous system to mature and for the brain to get used to the idea of walking on two legs. You may wonder what learning to walk has to do with meeting your weight-loss goals, but the effort and time it took you to walk really does mirror the effort and time it will take you to lose the weight you need to shed.

There are thousands, if not millions, of diet books and self-help guides available to us these days. Fads come and go. You've probably tried many of these strategies, and they have most likely failed to give you the results you have wanted. The question is, why has nothing really worked yet?

The problem—or problems, actually—is motivation, consistency, and perseverance, which are basically the keys to this whole plan. The fundamental core of most diets is not necessarily bad. The basic principle of eating and drinking fewer calories than you burn is a proven way of losing weight. Somewhere, there are people losing weight on almost any diet plan. They lose a bit, but when they stop the plan, they gain it all back and sometimes put on even more.

I have been practicing medicine for more than a decade. I have seen loved ones struggle with weight, and I have had my difficulties as well. I did not, however, struggle with weight when I was younger. My problems started because I was suffering from heart failure due to a congenital heart defect. I had put on more than seventy pounds in a few years, and I couldn't walk one hundred yards without taking a break. I was an army doctor, but I couldn't keep up with any of the other soldiers on runs or marches.

I had open-heart surgery in 2010 to fix the heart defect. Fortunately, the operation was a success, and I recovered. However, I was so severely deconditioned from years of inactivity that it took me years to bounce back and get out of my rut.

I have a soft spot in my heart for patients who are struggling with their weight and stuck in a rut. You may find yourself in a physical and/or an emotional slump for any number of reasons. Perhaps an emotional setback or (as in my case) a physical condition led you down this path. Either way, falling behind can be very demoralizing; we think that we are too far gone and wonder what the use is in trying. Making excuses also keeps us from making progress. It is easy to excuse why we eat this or that. Perhaps you have no time to prepare the right meals, and picking up dinner every night is more practical. Perhaps you think you can't exercise because you have sore knees or a bad back. Overcoming these barriers to sticking with a diet plan is not an easy hurdle to clear, but until you overcome it, nothing will change.

Advice for weight loss comes in two varieties: general and specific. The problem with general advice is that it is not a secret to anyone. For example, not eating junk food is a great piece of general advice—obvious, but not as easy as it sounds when you come down to it. What is junk food? What is not junk food? Is it really that clear cut? How much can I eat or should I eat? Unfortunately the general advice lacks specifics.

Specific advice, on the other hand, comes in every shape and size. You get it online, on TV, and from friends and family. Sometimes your doctor gives it to you, although we doctors are mostly good at the general advice like "Don't drink too much or smoke," and "Exercise and eat healthier."

Specific advice often contains only a fraction of what's needed to get the job done. For example, telling someone to eat one hundred grams of protein per day is not a bad piece of advice. The problem is that eating one hundred grams of protein by itself is one piece of a puzzle; without the other pieces, it will not do enough to help you lose weight. Now, I say "puzzle" because navigating the mountain of weight-loss advice can be like trying to put a puzzle together in the dark. It does seem so easy for some people to put things together and lose weight or stay slim. It can seem like luck, and unfortunately, it can be frustrating to others who feel like they will never figure it out. This probably sounds familiar. Don't feel bad or beat yourself up. It is normal to feel this way when facing a challenge that you seemingly can't overcome.

The key to success in surmounting these challenges is the main focus of this guide. You've read this far; just a little bit further and I'll let you in on my secrets for weight loss. I'll give you the same advice I give the patients I sit down with in my office. It *does* work. I've personally done it, and many of my patients and family members have turned their lives around using this information. You don't have to make an appointment with me to get this advice. You have all the tools you need in your hand right now.

Part I

Thinking about losing weight when you have a lot of it to lose can be troubling. It can seem like such a massive task that it appears almost impossible. Sure, if you start out today saying that you are going to lose one hundred pounds, you are probably going to fail—but not because of a specific diet or exercise regimen or lack of good intentions. You are more likely to fail because the goal can be overwhelming. You feel like you have bitten off more than you can chew, and keeping your eye on a goal that seems so far away is difficult.

Breaking large goals and tasks into smaller pieces makes them less intimidating and much more manageable. Your chances of success increase dramatically, especially if and when you get sidetracked. Often, things go well at first, but as soon as we encounter a setback, we tend to give up and throw away the small amount of work we have done.

Persistence and consistency are key. "Persistence" means refusing to give up. "Consistency" means doing the small steps over and over, day to day, so that they add up to a large goal over time. I discuss this in more detail in part II.

Because I am based in Canada, I like to use the analogy of walking to Florida. You shouldn't just say, "I am going to lose one hundred pounds," just as you wouldn't say, "I am going to walk to

Florida." Walking to Florida is nonsensical as a realistic goal. (If you live in or near Florida, substitute that state with somewhere thousands of miles away.) There is really no reason to walk to Florida—unless, of course, the zombie apocalypse has come and the last of our civilization is down there.

This walk to Florida is a mental exercise I use with patients to get their minds where they need to be to start the weight-loss journey. Unfortunately, losing weight can be a lot like that. Both goals are significant in their scope and impact on your life. They both take a lot of time, a lot of energy, and definitely some planning. Only persistence will get you there. If you don't keep walking, you will never get there.

Both of these goals are also significant achievements. I admit that you will end up with a better tan if you decide to walk to Florida, but dropping one hundred pounds will have more health benefits and make you feel immeasurably better. Not only does losing weight help you look better and boost your self-confidence, it also can have medical advantages. I have patients who come off their blood-pressure pills and diabetes medications once they shed weight. Perhaps this might be your motivation.

We have established that walking straight to Florida is a big task. If I were to ask you to get out of your chair and walk to the door of the examination room, there is a pretty good chance that you would. Walking from the chair to the door about ten feet away is a piece of cake, especially compared with walking the thousands of miles to Florida. If I ask you to walk from the examination room door to the front door of the office…another piece of cake. After that, you walk from the front door of the office to the end of the parking lot and then up to the road. Suddenly, you realize that once you reach the road, you have started your journey to Florida. You are actually on your way. Sure, you've only covered about one hundred feet, but that's one hundred feet fewer in your journey. If you walk one hundred feet toward Florida every day, eventually you are going to get there. If you stop walking, then obviously you will never make it.

By this point, you have probably realized what the title of this guide means. Take small steps toward Florida, and eventually you will get there. It is physically impossible to consistently walk toward Florida and actually not reach it, so long as you put in a little bit of daily effort. Keeping your mind on each day's little goal is what is most important. You cannot let yourself get sidelined by thinking about the entire journey to Florida. All you have to do is trust that if you stay on the road, you will get there eventually.

I have developed a diet and exercise plan I call the This Way diet because if you do your "walk to Florida" this way, you will achieve your goal. I am breaking down your steps to weight loss just as I have broken down your walk to Florida. There is no way you can fail as long as you follow a consistent and specific approach every day. You don't even have to think that much about it. Just do it. Remember, as long as you keep your feet moving on the road to Florida, you'll eventually arrive. I have tried to keep this guide as short as possible so you are not wasting time reading this book when you can be starting the plan and taking your life and health back.

Part II

I've presented the basic principle of motivation while using my This Way diet plan. Consistency and perseverance (or patience) are what you bring to the table. Again, consistency is sticking to the daily routine that you will adopt in your journey toward your goal. Consistency is what makes this plan work. I keep repeating this because it is really the only way you can reach a big goal.

Perseverance, or patience, is what keeps you going, especially when times get tough. This is an important point. Too often, unrealistic expectations make people give up on their goals because they feel like they will never achieve them. Setting up realistic expectations before beginning this program is very important as well. You may consider just doing the program consistently every day and seeing what happens without worrying about the time frame. That said, a good time frame for results is eighteen months. Sure, you will see results before then, but it took me about eighteen months from when I started my weight-loss journey till I could honestly look in the mirror and smile. (Unfortunately, I also had to buy a whole set of new clothes.)

There will be times when you stumble, cheat, or want to quit. It is precisely the analogy of walking to Florida that keeps you going when things get difficult. Say you get started, and you complete two weeks of the program (an excellent beginning, by the way). Then you stumble—skip a workout or two and cheat on your diet two days in a row. You're devastated; you think you've derailed your entire plan.

Then you think of your journey to Florida. You wouldn't throw away ten miles of progress just because you backtracked for a mile or rested for a couple of days; you would be throwing away the other nine miles you walked. You would take stock of where you are and realize that even though you have not been walking toward your goal for the last two days, you are still well on your way to Florida, as you have nine miles of walking under your belt. You're still pretty far from home. All you have to do is turn around and start moving your feet toward Florida again, and all is not lost. The same is true for your weight-loss program. You shouldn't throw away a week of effort just because of a day or two of cheating or abandoned workouts.

Part III

I developed the This Way plan after a lot of thought, analysis, and research, as well as a healthy dose of trial and error by those who followed the program. The ideas in this plan are based on biochemistry, physiology, medicine, and experience. It is important for me as a scientist to understand how the body metabolizes proteins, fats, and sugars. It is important for you to understand some basic physiological principles so that you can appreciate what it is you are doing to improve your health.

Everything has to make sense; otherwise, it is probably nonsense. My This Way weight-loss program consists of a logical approach to diet, portion-control macronutrient balance (protein, fat, carbohydrates), and exercise. The secret to this program is (you guessed it) consistency. I will outline the routine I have adopted and continue to follow every day. The nature of the program is that if you do things "This Way," you will succeed.

Table 1 outlines my daily routine, including sleep, diet, supplements, and exercise. It is the core of the program. This is what you will do to achieve your goals. This is your road to Florida. If you stick to this plan, you will get there.

My daily routine starts at 7:00 a.m. Of course, your start time may differ. Sticking to a routine is difficult if you are working shifts or if your life is very unpredictable. In this case, perhaps a first step

	The This Way Diet Program Daily Routine—Six Days Per Week (Table 1)
7:00 a.m.	Exercise 20 minutes—cycling/walking at a low to moderate pace
7:30 a.m.	Protein shake—16 oz. (500 ml) of milk with 2 scoops of This Way protein powder
11:00 a.m.	This Way protein bar (or substitute with veggies and nuts)
1:00 p.m.	This Way protein bar (or substitute with veggies and nuts)
5:00 p.m.	Large-leaf salad with 1–2 chicken breasts or other lean protein, dressing
7:00 p.m.	Exercise 20 minutes—cycling/walking at a low to moderate pace
7:30 p.m.	Small protein shake—8 oz. (250 ml) of milk with 1 scoop of This Way protein powder
10:00 p.m.	Bedtime—try to get a minimum of 8 hours of sleep

for you before starting the program will be to establish stability in your life to ensure success in the program. I had a patient who did work shifts but made an arrangement with her employer to work straight night shifts for six months so she could get into a routine and ensure success with the program. She went on to find another job that offered her the opportunity to work nine to five, and she has done quite well with the This Way diet. These kinds of major changes to your life are not necessary, but they might be something to consider if it means the difference between quitting the program and continuing toward your goal. If it were easy, we'd all be slim and in shape.

Research has shown that exercising before breakfast can burn up to 20 percent more fat than exercising after eating. Your muscles store sugar in the form of glycogen (organized sugar) so that they have something to use for energy when needed. If your muscles are full of sugar and you exercise, you don't need another source of energy to fuel your workout. But you want your body to be using the fat it has stored away in its main reserve of energy, like a bear that hibernates during the winter. The bear burns the body fat it accumulated in the fall for energy to stay alive until spring.

The problem with the fat we have on our bodies is that we continue to eat. In a perfect world, we would not eat for a couple of months, and our fat would melt away like a hibernating bear's. (Note that this is not a healthy way to lose weight, because as soon as you start eating again, your body will be in full crisis mode and will pack away as much fat as possible in anticipation for the next time you fast.)

Now picture the amount of sugar in your muscles after a whole night of fasting while you are sleeping. There isn't as much sugar available for continued exercise in the morning if you work out before breakfast. The result is that your body has to break down fat in order to feed the muscles you are using not only during exercise but also throughout your day. Exercising in the morning also revs up your metabolism (and therefore fat burning) for the rest of the day.

You'll notice in the daily routine that after your morning work-out, you will drink a protein shake for breakfast. The powder in this shake is a high-protein, low-fat, and low-carbohydrate powder. You can use my This Way Diet brand products, but you can substitute it with a different one. Keeping carbohydrates (or carbs) and fats low ensures that your body continues to use stored fat as its main source of energy after your workout and throughout your day. Adding milk to the protein powder instead of water does provide you with a bit of sugar and a bit of fat. (It also makes the shakes taste a heck of a lot better and therefore makes it more likely that you will stick to it.) Although you want to burn your fat stores, you need to consume some fat and some carbs to function, or else you end up in full starvation mode. You want to avoid this state of starvation because your body is programmed to freak out if this occurs. You want to give yourself just enough nutrients to avoid any drastic actions by your metabolism.

The other key to increasing and keeping your metabolism running quickly is to eat smaller regular meals. The easiest thing you can do to get fat is to eat only one or two large meals and do as little exercise as possible. In this program, we use the opposite strategy to get rid of the fat: eat multiple small meals and exercise regularly to burn off the sugars in your muscles. In the program, you increase your number of meals by spacing out the delivery of food and supplements to your system. Instead of having a large lunch, you will split up

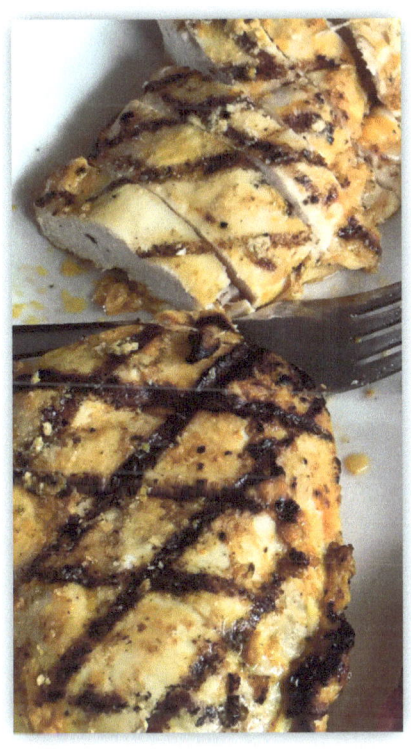

your midday meal into two separate servings of a protein bar. The protein bar serves two purposes: it controls the portion of food you deliver to your body so you don't overeat, and it keeps the carbs fairly low to force your metabolism to keep burning fat.

According to the daily routine in the program, dinner consists of a large, lettuce-based salad. I make mine with a lot of cucumbers, as they go a long way in filling me up and satisfying me for the evening. You add protein in the form of chicken, beef, pork, or fish (salmon, in my case). You could also use tofu as your evening protein. My typical salad consists of the lettuce, some celery, cucumbers, and carrot pieces all topped with a chicken breast or

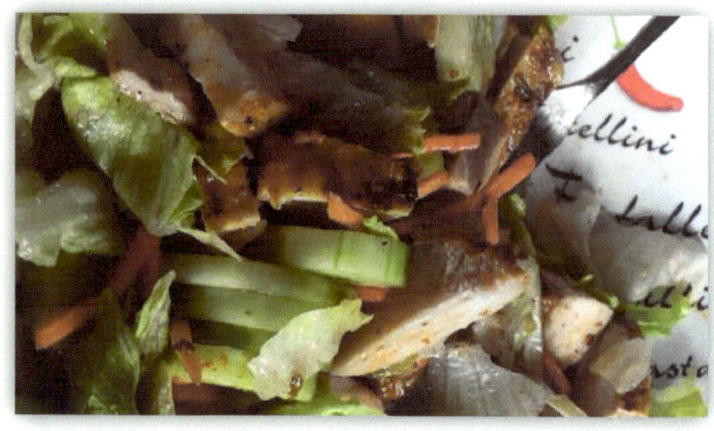

two and some bacon-ranch dressing, Greek feta dressing, or light raspberry dressing for taste. For ease of preparation, I often use a bagged salad from the grocery store. It is basically everything you need for your salad, chopped and ready to go in a small plastic bag. Don't underestimate the benefits of convenience when it comes to sticking to any program. The more difficult something is, the less likely you are to do it consistently over time.

I typically get a few things done around the house after dinner and then head downstairs to ride the stationary bike for another twenty minutes (as I did my first stationary bike workout at 7:00 a.m.) at about 7:00 p.m. The purpose of this evening exercise is to burn off some of the sugar in the muscles that has accumulated during the day and rev up the metabolism after having eaten a larger meal. When you eat a lot, your body goes into a "rest-and-digest" mode that, if not kept in check, will add to your waistline. Shutting off this rest-and-digest mode with stationary biking has worked like a charm for my patients and me.

After my evening exercise session, I try not to eat anything at all before bed. Unfortunately, I sometimes have a hard time sleeping when I am hungry, so the addition of a small protein shake after my workout can go a long way. I typically only make a half shake at night unless I am going crazy with hunger, then it's a full 16 oz shake. The real (read: medical) reason for the evening protein shake is to prevent your body from feeding on actual muscle tissue to make sugar overnight. This process is called gluconeogenesis, and your body will make sugar out of other things, like amino acids in protein and muscle tissue, if needed. Having enough protein in your stomach and your blood will keep muscle breakdown to a minimum.

We have come full circle in the daily routine of the program in that it is important to get sufficient sleep. Getting enough sleep is not just important to ensure that you will have the energy for your busy day and to avoid grumpiness; there is a medical reason as well. When our bodies are chronically under stress—for example, with regular lack of sleep—they go into a stress mode. The body produces a stress hormone called cortisol that has some nasty effects. Basically, what you need to know about cortisol is that it can raise your blood sugar and make your body accumulate fat. Cortisol also affects your immune system and your ability to fight off disease. It's the reason you catch every cold going around when you are under a lot of stress. You definitely want to avoid an increase in cortisol when you are trying to lose weight. Getting enough sleep at night and trying to minimize stress are the best ways to prevent increasing cortisol production. I really emphasize the need for sleep because it is a parameter that we can control, as opposed to other stresses in our lives that we often cannot.

Before we continue, it is important to mention that this program is for six days per week. That's right; you only have to abide by this program for six days out of the week, the seventh being your rest and cheat day. This is the day you will be looking forward to at first but may, believe it or not, actually come to loathe. I do have patients who chose not to have a cheat day, but I think including one is a healthy practice, especially at first. Having the cheat day to look forward to helps make the other six days manageable. But it is not a license to go crazy and make up for six days of restraint. It is a guilt-free day when you can indulge in some of the foods you love, keeping in mind that certain foods are worse than others. You will find over time that there are a lot of foods that you will no longer want to eat as often: fried foods will seem greasy, sweets will seem too sweet, and large meals will seem too large. This is not a bad thing at all!

Part IV

Now that we have reviewed the program and your new daily routine, I want to touch on some basic diet principles, taking into account biochemistry and physiology. I apologize if it gets a bit technical, but if you reread this part a few times, it won't seem as complicated. In fact, I will be simplifying some concepts, so don't get excited if you have a science background. This information doesn't quite match up 100 percent to what you know. In this case, the general idea is what's important, not the specifics.

We have all heard of carbs (that is, sugars and starches), proteins, and fats. One day in the news, carbs are bad for you, and another day it is the fats that are the devil. It is never the protein that is bad for you, and the reason has to do with how your body makes fat.

You will notice that protein is the central theme of this program's diet. Think of protein as the basic brick your body uses to make things, like hair, nails, muscle, and other tissues. Insulin is a hormone made of protein. Your body is a sneaky devil and can use protein for other things as well, such as making sugar (gluconeogenesis, from "gluco," meaning "sugar"; "neo," meaning "new"; and "genesis," meaning "creation"). The process of making sugar from protein is not a simple one, and your body prefers to use actual sugar rather than having to make it. That's one of the reasons I want you to eat enough protein: you have to eat something, or you will starve. Protein is not converted to sugar or fat as easily as actual sugar and fat. We want your body to work a little harder to feed itself and burn fat in the process. If you don't eat enough protein, your body will break down muscle to get the protein it needs.

Having plenty of protein available can also encourage your body to transform into a more athletic-looking one. An experiment involving native peoples in Canada (as shown in the CBC documentary *My Big Fat Diet*) showed that returning to a traditional diet of mostly protein and fat with very few carbs encouraged weight loss. Some people were even able to cease taking their diabetes medications as their metabolisms normalized.

Fats, on the other hand, do not play as many roles in the body for our purposes here. They are basically a way for your body to store energy for later when you have a lot that you don't need. When you move your arm or flex a muscle, you need energy, in the same way that a robot needs electricity to work its electric motors. I won't get into how energy is actually carried and used in the body, since it's a very complicated process. What is important to know is that fat is concentrated energy—lots of energy for its weight. It actually has so much energy in it that we use it to make candles. Fats (and their cousins, oils) are the best way for your body to store the energy it gets from food to use at a later time. Fat in the body is definitely a good thing, since you need fats to live, but as you know, too much of a good thing is bad.

Now we turn to sugar. Sugar is a chemical that is also rich in energy—not as rich as fat, but sugar's advantage is that it is very easy for your body to use as an energy source. Not much has to happen to sugar for your body to use it as energy. Unfortunately, if you eat more sugar than your body needs, the body fairly easily converts it to fat. Over time, if you don't burn off the energy (calories) that you have consumed, fat accumulates. The ease of use of sugar for energy is why you'll notice that the program in this guide is based on low carbs (low sugar).

I want to touch on another component that is perhaps the most crucial one, even though it's not really a nutrient: water. Water is important for obvious reasons. You need it to live—it makes up more than three-fourths of your body, it is the main constituent of blood and bodily fluids, and it is involved in your metabolism. This description is a very simplified version of water's role in the body, but I think it's necessary to appreciate how water plays a role in weight loss.

First, water plays a major part in weight loss because a lot of people confuse hunger with thirst. You could be thirsty (even chronically), and your mind might tell you to eat. You do get water from the foods you eat, so eating can often quench thirst, making you feel better. Over time, you associate that feeling of "hunger" (which is really thirst) with the need to eat. If you ensure that you are getting enough water in your system throughout the day, you're much less likely to feel that misguided hunger and chow down on empty calories.

A good place to start is about four regular-size water bottles (five-hundred-milliliter or sixteen-ounce bottles) per day, unless you have a medical condition where you have to restrict water intake. You will drink a lot of water in your shakes, but you will also need a bit more water than usual because you will be exercising. You can drink more than the minimum amount if you are thirsty and especially if the weather is hot.

The second property of water that is of interest to us in the context of weight loss is hydrolysis, or using water to break things down. This is really the key to setting up your fat-burning metabolism. When your body has to burn fat for energy—as it will because of the diet and exercise you will be doing—it has to break down the fat into smaller pieces to burn. Fat is stored in long chains of carbon that are sometimes called fatty acids.

These long chains of fat can be either trans fats (which are basically easily stackable bundles that can clog your arteries) or nontrans fats (or cis configuration, which is less stackable and consists of more fluid; it doesn't pile up or accumulate as much in your arteries). When your body wants to sever a piece of fat to use as energy, it uses a molecule of water to cut off a two-carbon piece. Think of it like this: if you have a lot of water in your system, your body will have an easier time reducing your fat reserves using this hydrolysis method. Without enough water, this process does not happen as easily and is slowed. That's why you need to make sure you drink enough water throughout your day.

Keeping these various macronutrients (protein, fat, sugar) in mind, I have avoided certain foods while doing this program mostly because of their sugar and sometimes their fat content. This is the part of the guide where you roll your eyes and more than likely start to curse my name. The foods to avoid while you are on this program are breads (all kinds, including crackers), pasta, rice, potatoes, sugars and syrups, cookies and cakes (obviously), anything fried, alcohol, and fruit.

"Fruit?" you say. I know; I am the devil. Fruit is supposed to be good for you. Well, it is, but I like to refer to it as "nature's candy." Fruits contain very simple sugars called fructose. The body uses fructose very easily for energy, and as a consequence, for also making fat. You may have heard of high-fructose corn syrup and that it isn't all that good for you, for the reason I just outlined. You can also think of fructose as a serving of white sugar when it comes to keeping your sugars in check.

Don't panic at this point, because the next section addresses the best part of this program…the cheat day!

Part V

I want to discuss this cheat day in the context of motivation. The whole premise of this program is that the journey to weight loss is like walking to Florida: it's a long road and a daunting task, but if you break it down into smaller goals and keep moving forward, you will get there.

When I unbutton my shirt, there is no giant "S" on my chest. I presume you don't have one, either, so jumping into this program twenty-four hours a day, seven days a week would be very, very difficult. I couldn't do it without a cheat day. The program itself is not easy. You will experience hunger, and it will take some time for you to get used to the feeling of never really being full. Anything worth doing is difficult, but I have found recharging my motivation by using a cheat day very useful. Cheating means not playing by the rules, and this day is exactly that. You play by the rules and stick to the program—exercise, protein shake, energy bar, energy bar, salad, meat, exercise, water, and sleep—six days per week. On the seventh day, you relax the diet.

When I say "relax the diet," I don't mean go completely crazy and hit the Chinese food buffet. I mean that this is the day when you can have the forbidden foods—bread, pasta, potatoes, and fruit. On my cheat days, I like to have a large berry bowl (strawberries, blueberries, raspberries) with Greek yogurt for breakfast, a sandwich like grilled cheese for lunch, and a nice bowl of spaghetti and meat sauce for dinner. Sometimes when I go out with friends, I will have pizza or a burger and fries for dinner. I often take the day off of exercise as well to let my muscles recover, and I sleep in a bit.

The hidden benefit to the cheat day is that it should introduce a little guilt into your mind. I always feel a little guilty after having had my cheat day, and it pushes me a little harder to get back on track the following day and for the rest of the week. I really feel at times that I have stepped off the road to Florida on my cheat day, and I am eager to get back on it because my goal of reaching Florida is getting closer and closer.

Conclusion

I am really happy that you have decided to read this guide and consider the program that I personally used to get into shape after my heart surgery. That is your first step on your personal road to Florida. Remember that the journey is long and difficult, but all you have to do is stay on the road, and you will get there. You will most likely have some setbacks during your journey and may even fall into a two-steps-forward-and-one-step-back pattern, but as long as you are still on the road to Florida, that's all that matters.

The secret to your success is not some magical recipe or concoction of fat burners and supplements. It is (say it with me) consistency. If you keep doing something, one day at a time, eventually it adds up, just like walking to Florida or saving money. The second secret is your new knowledge of your metabolism, including the importance of sleep to control cortisol levels, the importance of water in the hydrolysis of fats and suppressing appetite, the role of carbs (sugars) in making fat, and the timing of exercise to maximize the benefit to burning. Yes, putting them into action will take some time, but all you have to do is stick with the program, and you will get there.

I am excited for you and the changes that are to come. Read this guide more than once, and reread it when your motivation is low and you feel like giving up. You should be able to get through it easily in a day or a weekend. Copy or print the six-day program and put it on the fridge, your bathroom mirror, and your computer at work. When you see the simple plan and envision yourself walking on the road to Florida, your consistency and day-to-day determination will be rewarded with success in reaching your goal. Good luck, and let me know how you are doing! Also, check out my website for products and recommendations.

Twitter: @doctoruttley
Facebook.com/ThisWayDiet
Website: ThisWayDiet.com

Epilogue

I have made a few changes to the basic program as I have gotten into better and better shape. The program was very, very difficult for me in the beginning. It got easier as time went on, especially when I started to see and feel results. It took some time— about eighteen months, as I mentioned earlier—to get to where I wanted to be. Once I reached my goal, I developed new ones.

With my heart fixed and after a year and a half of exercise and dietary changes, I was feeling better than I ever had in my entire life. I was able to physically do things that were always very difficult for me. I had become so accustomed to pushing myself to stay with the program that eventually the exercise portion became too easy. I was starting to lose the feeling I once had after my workout. My body wasn't being challenged, and it was showing in the plateau I hit in my fitness level.

I made some changes in the duration and difficulty of exercise that I was doing. First, I doubled the exercise that I had become accustomed to doing every morning and evening. I now do forty minutes on the stationary bike every morning and every evening, and I have renewed that feeling I used to get after a workout. My fitness level has improved so much that it wasn't long before I was progressing in more challenging levels on the bike. Then I started doing push-ups and pull-ups in the morning. I also added leg lifts to my crunches.

Then I added a weight-lifting routine to my evening workout. I didn't want to sacrifice my fat-burning exercises, and the information available about weight lifting and cardio exercises was confusing and conflicting. I decided to continue with my forty minutes on the stationary bike and then do weights. I had three major body parts that were very lacking: shoulders, legs, and arms. It wasn't until I lost a lot of weight that I could really see the weaknesses in my physique. For years I was overweight, and now that I had fixed that problem, I needed to touch up a few other areas. I had not lifted weights in years, so I started very light and worked my way up in both weight and frequency over time. It does no good to injure yourself by trying to do too much too soon. Below is an updated table of the advanced program I do today.

Another difference with what I am doing now is that I don't seem to need an all-out cheat day anymore. I have seen such a transformation in my body that I consciously continue to make smarter food selections even on my cheat day. It is as though the closer I get to my ultimate goal, and in an attempt to maintain the results of eighteen months of hard work, the less I let completely loose. Admittedly, there are weeks when I don't even need a cheat day, but I always take a rest day no matter what. On the cheat day, I relax my midday meal (and actually eat something more substantive), but I usually continue having my shake in the morning. Dinner consists of a protein (chicken, steak, or pork) with a side of salad, which basically is just a variation of a large salad with a protein on it.

It is so satisfying to have reached my weight-loss goal. For me, the ultimate feeling is when I go try on new clothes. Having

	The This Way Diet Advanced Program Daily Routine— Six Days Per Week (Table 2)
7:00 a.m.	Exercise 40 minutes—cycling, 60 ab crunches, 30 leg lifts, 30 push-ups, 10 pull-ups
8:00 a.m.	Protein shake—16 oz. (500 ml) of milk with 2 scoops of This Way protein powder
11:00 a.m.	This Way protein bar and some fruit (e.g., an apple, pineapple pieces, or melon)
1:00 p.m.	This Way protein bar (or substitute with veggies and nuts)
5:00 p.m.	Large-leaf salad with 1–2 chicken breasts or other lean protein on the side (steak or pork chops), dressing on the salad. Add a baked potato or some rice if too hungry.
7:00 p.m.	Exercise 40 minutes—cycling or running on treadmill (2 minutes walking, 2 minutes running)
7:40 p.m.	Weight lifting (3–4 days per week, not on running days); either shoulders (3 exercises), arms (2 exercises for both biceps and triceps), or legs (leg presses, lunges, dead lifts, calf extensions)
8:30 p.m.	Protein shake—16 oz. (500 ml) of milk with 2 scoops of This Way protein powder—only on weight-lifting days or if too hungry to sleep
10:00 p.m.	Bedtime—try to get a minimum of 8 hours of sleep

everything fit and not being embarrassed to step out of the changing room and stand in front of the mirror is priceless. Stick with this program, and I have no doubts at all that in no time you will feel the same way.

www.ingramcontent.com/pod-product-compliance
Lightning Source LLC
Chambersburg PA
CBHW050858290526
45792CB00002B/647